Managing Fibromyalgia

Causes, Symptoms and
Treatment Options
To
Reduce the Pain

RON KNESS

Copyright © 2017 Ron Kness
All rights reserved.

**ISBN-13: 978-1544093291
ISBN-10: 1544093292**

Contents

Disclaimer

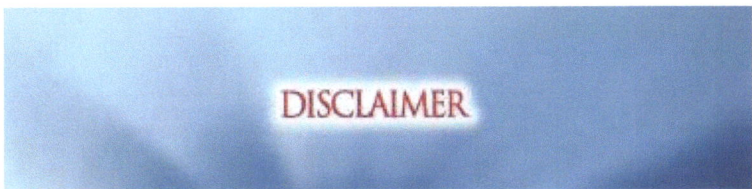

This publication is for informational purposes only and is not intended as medical advice. Medical advice should always be obtained from a qualified medical professional for any health conditions or symptoms associated with them. Every possible effort has been made in preparing and researching this material. We make no warranties with respect to the accuracy, applicability of its contents or any omissions.

See your healthcare professional before starting any diet, health or exercise program!

Introduction

INTRODUCTION

Fibromyalgia is a truly insidious condition. While most who suffer with it say they would not wish it upon anyone, in truth many wish that others could experience what they do, if only for a short time.

The condition is a life sentence, there is no cure. The symptoms can be general and diverse, but mostly revolve around persistent and recurring pain. There is rarely an obvious cause, which leaves many sufferers believing others see them as hypochondriacs.

Fibromyalgia can be difficult to diagnose. In the past, some doctors were reluctant to make the diagnosis. Before attributing a patient's symptoms to the condition a doctor must rule out other conditions which have similar or overlapping symptoms.

This publication hopes to provide understanding of the condition to those who don't suffer from fibromyalgia (but may know someone who does) and to provide hope and assistance to those who do.

Although there is currently no cure for the condition, its effects can be greatly reduced by many different means.

What Is Fibromyalgia?

WHAT IS FIBROMYALGIA

Fibromyalgia is defined as a chronic disorder which negatively affects the mind and body. It can devastate an active lifestyle and is characterized by overwhelming fatigue, muscle and joint pain, and much more.

The exact medical translation of the term, fibromyalgia, is "pain in the muscles, ligaments and tendons." However, if you suffer from fibromyalgia, you will know that this definition falls far short of explaining the range of effects the condition causes you.

Difficult to Diagnose

Searching for a diagnosis and relief from the symptoms of fibromyalgia can be frustrating and you may experience a long journey of medical tests to rule out other conditions such as lupus, thyroid and arthritis.

The pain and other symptoms of fibromyalgia may vary at times – even causing you to experience energy and freedom from pain one day but complete lack of motivation, plus extreme pain the next day.

The variability in type and frequency of symptoms has made effective diagnosis and study very elusive. This has led to many instances of misdiagnosis.

When health professionals have not managed to connect the dots, the symptoms have often been attributed to alternative conditions, or the symptoms treated in isolation. Many sufferers report years of condescending attitudes from doctors and even loved ones, hinting at hypochondria due to not having a "real" diagnosed condition.

Debilitating and Far-reaching

The chronic pain and fatigue caused by this disorder may cause some people to withdraw from activities they used to enjoy and failure to work at the pace they need.

Many who suffer with the condition lose their jobs and are unable to properly care for children or take care of other normal and on-going responsibilities.

Physical repercussions of fibromyalgia may include irritable bowel syndrome and overactive bladder – making it even more difficult to leave home or socialize with others.

Mental and Emotional Health Affected

Depression and anxiety may often accompany the symptoms of fibromyalgia, especially if the person feels emotionally unsupported. The domino effect of this heinous disorder can cause a person to give up on ever enjoying a normal life again.

Fibromyalgia isn't new. In fact, it's been around for centuries and perhaps diagnosed as rheumatism or other diseases of the joints and muscles.

The medical community has been slow to accept the disorder as a viable state of chronic pain originating in the body's tissues, but most have recently come around to the fact that fibromyalgia is a distinct medical syndrome.

Women Most Often Affected by Fibromyalgia

Fibromyalgia is complex – affecting more women than men. Children can also suffer from the disorder. It can affect people of all ages, backgrounds and body structure. Intensity of pain may vary from one person to the other and be more intense some days than others.

The disorder of fibromyalgia continues to confound the medical community in many ways, but hope for relief of the pain and suffering it causes is strong for the coming years due to increasing awareness of the extent of the condition.

New scientific research is reducing the stigma of chronic pain and identifying more ways to help sufferers regain their quality of life without turning to opioids or invasive surgery.

Incurable, but Manageable

Although fibromyalgia is incurable, it can be effectively managed. Self-management strategies such as meditation, exercise and medications may help to relieve some of the symptoms of fibromyalgia and get your life back on track.

What Causes Fibromyalgia?

WHAT CAUSES FIBROMYALGIA

The possible causes and risk factors of fibromyalgia are as varied as the symptoms of the disorder. All the theories and explanations are yet unproven, but there is some research to indicate that certain theories seem more valid than others.

Age and Gender a Factor

For example, hormonal disruptions (such as menopause in middle-aged women) are widely believed to be a factor in developing the disease later in life. This is statistically supported, as this demographic has the highest amount of those affected by symptoms of fibromyalgia.

Fibromyalgia is much more common in women and women experience wide-ranging hormonal changes during menopause. Women who have fibromyalgia also have low levels of the human growth hormone, which may cause muscle pain.

Mental Issues More a Symptom Than a Cause

Anxiety and depression also have strong links to fibromyalgia, but are no longer considered causes of the disorder. However, chronic pain suffered during severe fibromyalgia episodes may lead to feelings of anxiety and low grade depression.

There may also be a genetic tendency toward developing fibromyalgia. Some genes may cause a more intense reaction to certain stimuli than others, causing one person to perceive pain while the next person would not.

Physical and Emotional Stress Probable Triggers

Many medical professionals now believe that stress or some type of muscle trauma (minor damage) may initially trigger the vicious cycle of pain and extreme fatigue that sufferers are all too familiar with.

Other theories indicate that fibromyalgia may result from a variety of factors including emotional or physical stress, low levels of serotonin and sleep disorders.

Many have speculated that a person's inability to produce natural pain blockers (endorphins) or elevated levels of the chemical termed "substance P" may also be causes.

Hormonal Influences

Substance "P" is released by the body in response to stressors. It triggers hormonal responses including a heightened pain response to stimulate us to move away from danger.

Like many of our "fight or flight" hormones, substance "P" would have been critical to our evolutionary survival.

However, today our stresses are more often triggered by emotional factors than physical life and death situations. It is theorized that persistently elevated levels of "P" will therefore cause a corresponding heightened and prolonged pain response.

Associated Risk Factors

Risk factors for fibromyalgia are almost as varied as the causes. Some women who suffer from lupus, arthritis or similar autoimmune disease may develop other symptoms associated with fibromyalgia, but most develop the disorder without experiencing another disease.

There is a history of some fibromyalgia sufferers developing the disorder after experiencing trauma to the brain or spinal cord. Car accidents may lead to the diagnosis if pain and emotional trauma was endured.

The bottom line is that there seems to be no single reason that a person develops fibromyalgia. That's why it's so difficult for doctors to diagnose.

If you suspect you have fibromyalgia, keep a record of your feelings and pain flare ups so you can discuss them and point out the reasons for your suspicions.

More scientific research and a better understanding among health care providers about the causes and risk factors of fibromyalgia are leading to more effective treatments and methods of managing this devastating disorder.

Fibromyalgia Symptoms

FIBROMYALGIA SYMPTOMS

Although men and children can suffer from fibromyalgia, the disorder is most common among women, who represent 80 to 90 percent of those affected, and most are diagnosed sometime during middle age.

You are more likely to develop fibromyalgia if you have a close relative with the disorder – or if you've been in predicaments involving car accidents, repetitive injuries such as back problems or infections and other illnesses.

Symptoms Parallel Other Conditions

One of the reasons that fibromyalgia is so difficult to diagnose is that it mimics so many other diseases' and disorders' symptoms.

Some fibromyalgia symptoms parallel other diseases and disorders to such an extent that it's difficult to acquire a diagnosis without undertaking medical tests to rule out other conditions.

Rheumatoid arthritis, arthritis and lupus may mimic fibromyalgia in many ways, or at least share some the same symptoms, making it even more difficult to make an accurate diagnosis.

Generalized Pain

Pain may occur anywhere over the entire body, making it difficult for medical professionals to diagnose the underlying cause. Especially vulnerable to pain are tender areas of the body such as the legs, arms, hips, neck and shoulders. When pressure is put on these points, severe pain may occur, similar to pressing on a deep bruise.

Mental and Emotional Effects

Cognitive problems (also called "fibro fog") may occur with those suffering from fibromyalgia. Many sufferers of fibromyalgia become depressed or suffer severe anxiety as performing every day activities becomes increasingly difficult.

Headaches, restless leg syndrome and numbness of the hands and feet can also contribute to the list of symptoms.

Pain and Fatigue

Chronic pain and extreme fatigue are the most common complaints of fibromyalgia sufferers. Muscle spasms often accompany the fatigue and pain so that sleep or engaging in any activity becomes a major problem.

This can lead to sleep deprivation and inability to concentrate or perform day to day chores or engage socially with others.

Compromised Immune System

Over time, this combination of physical and mental symptoms can wear the patient down, leading to emotional issues such as depression.

The chronic nature of the condition can also negatively impact the immune system, making the body less able to defend itself against environmental effects.

This in turn means increased susceptibility to things like cold and flu viruses, plus increased duration of its effects. Also, of course, due to the insidious effects of fibromyalgia, the pain, discomfort and feelings of lethargy of subsequent infections are more strongly experienced.

Sensitivity to a Wide Range of Stimuli

Sensitivity to touch is also a major complaint of those with the disorder. Even a light blanket might feel like a heavy weight on top of you.

This is called hyperesthesia – a cousin of another symptom called hyperalgesia, which is an increase in pain perception characterized by feeling pain from a slight bump which may have occurred days or even weeks later.

Sensitivity to bright lights, certain smells (especially from chemicals) and loud noises can also trigger headaches or other reactions from those suffering with fibromyalgia. Cold and heat can also be more vividly experienced.

Almost all environmental stimuli can be greatly exacerbated by the condition.

A layman's summary might describe fibromyalgia as causing hypersensitivity to most areas of existence. For the sufferer, this translates to unreasonable and persistent feelings of pain and discomfort.

Fibromyalgia Tender Points

FIBROMYALGIA AND TENDER POINTS

A person who suffers from fibromyalgia may feel that the entire body is a tender point because of the extreme pain that radiates through their muscles and joints. Actually, there are 9 specific pairs (18 points in all) that are painful when pressure is applied. These points may radiate pain over the entire body.

A Primary Diagnostic Tool

The tender points are localized around (not within) joints in the body and usually just beneath the surface of the skin. When pressed with a finger on these points, pain results. While the painful area may be perceived by the sufferer as being inflamed, when the site is examined no inflammation is found to exist.

Confirming Symptoms Required for Diagnosis

Even though the tender points of fibromyalgia are predictable, the disorder cannot be conclusively diagnosed by relying on that examination alone.

Other symptoms that will assist a doctor to confirm a diagnosis may include extreme fatigue, depression, irritable bowel syndrome, sleep disorders and others.

When undertaking an examination to test for tender points response, doctors will also test control points on the patient. These are points on the body which usually won't cause the pain reaction that occurs to the tender points of the fibromyalgia sufferer.

Treatment for Pain

The treatment for tender point pain that radiates throughout the body may be multi-faceted and extend beyond remedies that only focus on the physical aspects. Some people respond to anti-depressants while others may react better to stress management such as exercise and rest.

Alternative Remedies

Alternative medical treatments can also be effective methods to manage fibromyalgia pain. For example, therapeutic massage can help the muscles and soft tissues by simulating them to relieve tension and stress.

This can assist with the pain the specific tender points and also the referred pain. This referred pain presents as general, all-over pain and is the bane of the fibromyalgia patient.

Learning to reduce your stress and control your stress response is important after a diagnosis of fibromyalgia. Rest and relaxation can ease the everyday tension and keep you from becoming extremely fatigued – one of the tender point pain triggers.

Avoid Environmental Extremes

Where possible, avoid extreme cold or humidity. These factors can greatly affect the intensity of pain at the tender points of your body. Also, these conditions combined with your possibly diminished immune system increase your risk of viral infection, which again, increases your pain levels.

While rest is important, you don't want to live a completely sedentary lifestyle. That makes the muscles and joints more tender and painful when they are put to use. Engage in exercises that aren't overly strenuous but will still benefit your breathing and your muscle tone.

Work Around Your Condition

Determine which times of day your tender points are manifesting the most pain and as much as possible make plans to rest during those times. Perhaps, soak in a warm bath or Jacuzzi or use those times for meditation or complete relaxation.

Keep in mind that pain from the tender points must be present for more than three months before a diagnosis of fibromyalgia can be considered. Consider keeping a log or diary of your pain levels and variables such as weather, ambient temperature, foods eaten and any events which invoke an emotional response.

Be Part of the Solution

Help is available and can make a distinct difference to your quality of life. However, try not to leave finding relief from the pain of tender points solely to your doctor.

Your ability to provide specific rather than general answers (from your records) to your doctor's questions will help your doctor help you.

Fibromyalgia and Depression

FIBROMYALGIA AND DEPRESSION

If you've been diagnosed with fibromyalgia, it's important to realize that the disorder affects more than muscles and tender points. Not only does it cause pain, but eventually it challenges your entire way of life – feelings, attitude and other emotions.

It would be almost impossible not to suffer from some level of depression when suffering from fibromyalgia. The connection between fibromyalgia and depression is very real. Studies show that those with fibromyalgia are about three times more prone to depression than someone without the devastating disorder.

No one knows the exact reason for the link. It could be that the same changes or abnormalities in the nervous system and brain chemistry which make a person more sensitive to pain also causes them to be more prone to depression.

Living with Fibromyalgia

Even if and when this is not the case, the simple reality of having to live as a fibromyalgia sufferer is certain to cause intense feelings of negative emotion. Feeling sad or low is a normal reaction to the pain and other symptoms of fibromyalgia.

It is very difficult to maintain a positive attitude when you go to bed at night in pain, wake in pain, and know that there will possibly be more pain during the day, all seemingly without apparent cause. It is disheartening having to rely on pain relievers just to make it through the day.

It is even more distressing when the wants of children and spouse cannot be met to their or your expectations.

Fibromyalgia sufferers often experience feelings of wanting to curl up in a ball and wish the world would go away. Knowing it won't and they must try to work through their physical pain and mental distress drags them further down emotionally.

For a fibromyalgia sufferer already dealing with low energy levels and loss of pleasure in formerly enjoyable activities, this chronic sadness can manifest in feelings of guilt, worthlessness and even thoughts of death.

Recognizing Depression

Those who suffer from fibromyalgia may or may not know they're suffering from depression, which is a condition itself. They may characterize their feelings as simply being overwhelmed by their circumstances.

Some may realize something is wrong, but may think that the decreased energy, inability to concentrate, irritability and anxiety is more physical than mental.

The constant stress of living with symptoms of fibromyalgia can cause your nervous system to become overloaded with a range of overwhelming feelings including anxiety, anger and guilt. Ultimately this can and very often results in depression.

Need for Action to Deal with Depression

It is important that you gain control over symptoms of depression associated with fibromyalgia. Most people diagnosed with depression are encouraged to look for the cause of their depression – if you have been diagnosed with fibromyalgia you already know the cause.

Feelings of depression are valid symptoms of fibromyalgia. When discussing your range of symptoms with your health care provider don't gloss over them, or focus only on the physical effects.

This will help the doctor to better suggest methods of treatment that are right for you.

The method of controlling or reducing depression symptoms you choose may include antidepressants, or more natural methods of control such as exercise, meditation, positive changes in diet and other alternative techniques.

Biofeedback, acupuncture, meditation and light exercises can help lighten your mood and lessen your pain.

Although there's no specified cure for the fibromyalgia disorder, the symptoms, including depression, can be treated successfully.

It's vital that you strive to find a way to manage the symptoms before you begin a downward spiral which can affect your entire life, including relationships and career.

Take steps to deal with and find effective means to combat your feelings of depression if you've been diagnosed with fibromyalgia. Don't simply accept that this is your lot without making efforts to improve your quality of life.

There are treatments available which can greatly reduce the symptoms and help you enjoy life once again.

Fibromyalgia and Weight Gain

FIBROMYALGIA AND WEIGHT GAIN

It is especially frustrating for the person suffering from fibromyalgia to have the added tendency to gain weight. Weight management is an effort for almost anyone, for fibromyalgia sufferers the challenges are greatly increased.

Compounding Factors

There are several factors which may contribute to weight gain among fibromyalgia sufferers. Side effects from prescribed medications and pain that prevents strenuous exercise can sabotage any efforts to keep the weight off while still fighting fibromyalgia symptoms.

Medications used to treat symptoms of fibromyalgia definitely play a role in weight gain. Antidepressants are the worst culprits, but other medications may also contribute to unwanted pounds from increased body fat.

Weight gain in someone diagnosed with fibromyalgia can often be partly attributed to a decreased metabolism, increase in appetite, hormone deficiency and fluid retention. If you also suffer from depression, which is likely, the antidepressants will play a role in weight gain.

Even when you do eat less, you may notice little difference in weight – simply because of the other changes happening within your body. However, this can be mitigated by choices in the types of food consumed.

Hormone imbalances are prevalent for those who suffer from fibromyalgia. Growth hormone, thyroid, serotonin and cortisol level fluctuations cause the body's metabolism to slow and there may also be insulin problems. These issues may cause the body to store excess fat.

One common factor is a lack of quality sleep, or simply always feeling fatigued. It is difficult to get a good night's sleep with fibromyalgia pain and other symptoms. This leads to a slower metabolism and increased appetite, especially for sugar and high-carb foods.

These are the food type that our brains have us unconsciously crave when tired or depressed – exactly the common circumstances of a fibromyalgia sufferer. They are also the foods that not only most contribute to increased boy fat, they also encourage continued eating, as they do not help us feel full or satisfied.

Exercise

Decreased activity due to pain may also contribute to an increase in weight as you less efficiently burn the calories you consume. With fibromyalgia, it's not always practical to suggest exercise as a way to reduce weight.

The pain associated with the disorder can make it difficult to engage in exercises such as aerobic and other fat-burning methods.

However, although exercise is very beneficial, diet is a much bigger factor in weight gain, so don't let reduced exercise become an excuse. Focus on food choices and portion sizes instead.

Good Diet Essential

The best way to control your weight after a fibromyalgia diagnosis is through a well thought out diet plan. High protein - low carbohydrate plans are best. Lean meats, some dairy, soy and legumes are good sources of protein.

It is important to limit consumption of sweets, breads, pastas, rice, potatoes, soft drinks and alcohol.

Only eat until you're full – not stuffed. Eat slowly and chew your food well. Eat several small meals per day rather than three large ones. This will help reduce snacking and keep your metabolism on a steady path to reduce the highs and lows you may feel during the day.

Mindfully choosing better foods, especially quality protein foods, is a necessary part of not just weight loss, but also reducing the negative effects of fibromyalgia.

Many sufferers have noted improvements after making positive dietary changes. This does require effort on the part of the patient, but the results are worth it.

Before making major changes to your diet or exercise plan, be sure to discuss it with your doctor. Consider asking about possible testing for such maladies as hormone deficiency, thyroid problem, yeast or hypoglycemia.

These medical problems also cause weight gain and the symptoms may mimic those of fibromyalgia.

Fibromyalgia Diet

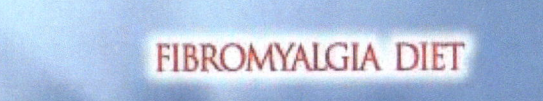

If you are one of the millions who suffer fatigue and muscle pain from fibromyalgia, you're likely grasping for ways to help reduce or relieve the debilitating symptoms.

Although a specific diet plan isn't the total solution to relieving pain or other symptoms, research indicates that there are certain foods which can reduce the effects for some people.

Most of the research has been gathered by patients who report how consuming and more importantly avoiding certain foods has played a role in alleviating particular symptoms of fibromyalgia.

There is increasing awareness that diet is a bigger factor in human health than previously given credit for. We know that food can make us feel up or down and affect our energy levels. Those with fibromyalgia may have sensitivities which magnify those feelings.

For example, MSG, gluten, eggs, dairy and preservatives may negatively affect a person who suffers from the fibromyalgia disorder.

Keep a Food Journal

The best thing you can do yourself before tweaking your diet to help your symptoms is to pay close attention to what you are eating and how you feel afterwards. Keep a diet journal and jot down your mood and pain level a few hours after eating and you'll soon get a picture of which foods are helping and which are aggravating your symptoms.

You may notice that your joint pain worsens or you have headaches and severe fatigue after consuming a certain food. Your journal will make it easier to see patterns and you can then adjust your diet accordingly.

It can be very empowering and even exciting to discover correlations between specific food items and the responses they cause.

Elimination Diet

It may be helpful to try the elimination challenge diet, which means that you stop eating a particular food you suspect you have a sensitivity to.

For example, irritable bowel syndrome is a common problem of fibromyalgia sufferers and diet often plays a part in the irritation.

Stop eating the food for six to eight weeks and see how you feel. Spicy foods, those which contain gluten and dairy products are often culprits of irritable bowel syndrome, so try eliminating those in the beginning of your research.

Many report a lessening of bloating, fatigue and constipation when these types of foods are removed from their diet.

Be careful about eliminating foods from your diet that may contain needed nutrients. You may want to consult with a dietitian to plan an elimination diet to be sure you don't further harm your immune system and cause more problems.

Foods to Overcome Fatigue

Some foods can be added to your diet to help fight the fatigue experienced with fibromyalgia. Eating small meals throughout the day may help as can protein snacks to boost your energy level as well as helping you avoid feeling hungry.

Supplements may also help your fibromyalgia symptoms. Discuss any supplements you're considering with your health care provider as some may interact with other medications you may be taking.

Lifestyle Changes Can Help

Make positive changes to your diet and experience the ongoing benefits. Learning which foods to avoid is a big step in reducing the effects of your condition.

Also, keep in mind that your entire lifestyle affects your symptoms, not only directly, but also in how it affects your eating patterns and behaviors.

Therapies such as massage, deep-breathing, yoga and meditation can be combined with a healthy diet plan to give you the best quality of life you can experience in spite of fibromyalgia.

How to Manage Fibromyalgia

HOW TO MANAGE FIBROMYALGIA

There is no known cure for fibromyalgia. For those diagnosed with the condition, treatment comes down to learning how to best manage its effects. Ideally this means reducing both the incidence and intensity of symptoms, foremost of which is usually physical pain.

There are other symptoms, but these are mostly caused or worsened by the ongoing struggle with pain. Those who suffer from fibromyalgia often additionally suffer from inflammation causing tenderness, chronic fatigue, lack of concentration and stiffness.

The persistent and ongoing nature of these symptoms can very often result in varying degrees of mental and emotional problems. These issues can then add to the mix of symptoms, compounding and worsening the apparent effects, and reducing the ability to cope.

Diagnosis and Cause

It's not easy to diagnose fibromyalgia, but most physicians use a method of noting reaction to 11 to 18 tender points of the body as a primary diagnostic tool.

Patient demographics are an indicator, as many more women than men contract the condition, increasingly as they get older.

Although fibromyalgia doesn't have a single cure, treatments and remedies do exist which will help you manage the pain, depression, stress and anxiety associated with the disorder.

Addressing the root causes of your instance of fibromyalgia is the key to finding the most effective solutions to treat the symptoms. For example, an intolerance to gluten, stress (either physical or mental) and chronic inflammation may trigger or contribute to many of the symptoms.

Treatment of Fibromyalgia Symptoms

There are a variety of effective approaches and remedies available, and those you choose will depend on what your specific symptoms are.

Conventional drugs may be prescribed to lessen the symptoms, especially for pain relief, but these can potentially cause severe side effects – so, it's best to search for possible natural remedies to relieve the symptoms.

Massage therapy, biofeedback, acupuncture and chiropractic manipulation are considered effective management techniques for fibromyalgia sufferers. All of them are safe and can provide some relief for even the most traumatic pain and anxiety.

Topical and Oral Remedies

Applying a cream called Capsaicin (derived from a pepper plant) is said to be a natural pain reliever. It stimulates "substance P," a body chemical which helps relieve pain temporarily.

Melatonin hormone therapy is known to help promote sleep. Lack of sleep is a common complaint among fibromyalgia sufferers and melatonin in pill form may also help reduce chronic pain.

Dietary Changes

Changes to your diet such as adding anti-inflammatory nutrients may help muscle and joint pain.

Those who suffer from fibromyalgia may have nutritional deficiencies such as magnesium. Magnesium is essential for allowing the muscles to relax and many people in western societies are deficient in this vital mineral.

You can choose to take magnesium supplements or add such foods as flax and pumpkin seeds, almonds, halibut and black beans to your diet.

Quercetin (an element found in red onion and black and green teas) can naturally help to reduce inflammation in the body. Omega-3 fats such as those in fish oil can also reduce inflammation.

Stress can be a Cause and a Symptom

If incidences of stress bring on fibromyalgia symptoms, then continually only using pain-blocking medication won't be the most effective resolution, although it is an understandable and commonly used solution. Stress increases cortisol levels, which in turn stimulates inflammation markers and causes pain.

When stress is a known trigger, to achieve a reduction in occurrences it will be necessary to avoid or reduce the stressors, or learn to deal better with the stress, thereby reducing its impact and subsequent triggering of fibromyalgia symptoms.

There are many effective methods for reducing stress and anxiety by utilizing natural relaxation methods.

Reducing the effects of fibromyalgia involves firstly determining the triggers, then reducing the impact of symptoms using a combination of available solutions.

Natural Remedies for Fibromyalgia

NATURAL REMEDIES FOR FIBROMYALGIA

Healthy Lifestyle Essential

For all sufferers, regardless of individual symptomatic differences, seeking to achieve an overall healthy lifestyle should be an ongoing goal.

The last thing a fibromyalgia patient needs is their fragile immune system further compromised by an influx of toxins, either from their diet or environmental influences.

Various medications can be prescribed by your health care provider to lessen pain and other symptoms, but a more holistic and natural approach is now gaining popularity.

Although pharmaceutical options such as antidepressants, anti-inflammatories and other non-steroidal drugs and pain killers are commonly relied upon, long-term use invariably has unwanted side effects.

Even ubiquitous over-the-counter analgesics can cause organ damage or diminished function when used for long periods. Wherever possible, where a more natural or drug-free option exists, it is in your interest to at least try it.

Reducing Pain

If muscle spasms or aches is one of your main symptoms, taking a warm bath before you go to bed can provide some relief. You may need a prescription for muscle relaxers, but if you can reduce the severity of the pain and discomfort with baths, massage and gentle exercises, it will be much better for your overall, and especially long-term, health.

When tender points, fatigue and deep muscle pain seems to be your worst symptom, try exercise. It may seem contradictory to keeping pain at bay, but exercises such as swimming, yoga, stretches and tai chi are low impact and have been shown to reduce pain from fibromyalgia.

Other Natural Options

It may help to manage irritable bowel syndrome (IBS) by consuming more fiber in your diet. Even though high fiber may cause other symptoms such as bloating and gas, high-fiber foods such as beans, fruits and vegetables are known as effective in treating IBS when consumed gradually over a period of several weeks.

Check into the possibility of biofeedback treatments to ease fibromyalgia pain and stress. This is a mind and body relaxation method which uses electronics to measure various stress responses.

You can then use that information to control your level of relaxation and subsequently reduce pain and anxiety.

Acupuncture, the ancient Chinese method of relieving pain and restoring the flow of energy in the body, is effectively used as an alternative treatment for fibromyalgia.

Acupuncture involves stimulating certain points of the body by inserting very slim needles just below the skin.

Improving Sleep

Sleep disorders are a huge part of the problem for those living with fibromyalgia. Maintaining a healthy bedtime routine can improve sleep quantity and quality, which will provide many positive flow-on effects. This routine should include striving for complete silence, darkness and peace in the bedroom and using techniques such as warm baths and massage just before bed.

Healthy eating, exercise, massage, deep breathing techniques and reducing toxic inputs is a good start for managing symptoms of fibromyalgia naturally.

Sufferers wish there was a magic pill or remedy for the symptoms, however the reality is you can live your healthiest life by as much as possible utilizing the natural remedies that work best for you.

Be sure to research and discuss with your doctor possible negative interactions with other medications you may be taking before using natural remedies for relieving pain and other symptoms of fibromyalgia.

Natural Supplements for Fibromyalgia

NATURAL SUPPLEMENTS FOR FIBROMYALGIA

Using natural supplements to relieve pain and other symptoms of fibromyalgia has proven beneficial for many who suffer from the disorder. One of the suspected causes of fibromyalgia in many patients is a deficiency of one or more nutrients in the body.

Fibromyalgia also causes depletion of nutrients, so personally researching and testing natural supplements can be a good way to find your own solutions to help diminish the symptoms.

Do Your Own Research

There is much information both online and in books about which supplements work and which may harm your health when taken with other medications or supplements. Use the experience of those who have already experimented and had satisfactory results.

Be smart about taking any supplements to relieve fibromyalgia symptoms. Be systematic in using any supplements and monitor and record dosage and subsequent effects.

Don't experiment with radical dosages. If in any doubt, consult with your doctor about the correct dosage or any negative interaction the supplements may have with prescribed medications.

Supplements to Consider

Low Vitamin D and magnesium levels have been found to be prominent in those sufferers of fibromyalgia. A deficiency in either or both will almost certainly cause or worsen fibromyalgia symptoms.

Vitamin D (the sunshine vitamin) may be effective in reducing nerve and muscle spasms of those with the disorder. Taking a vitamin D supplement, especially for those with limited sun exposure, can help reduce pain and fight the fatigue commonly associated with the fibromyalgia.

Magnesium is essential for helping muscles to relax; a deficiency is known to contribute to muscle cramps. Usage has been shown to significantly improve fibromyalgia symptoms.

Magnesium is found in cocoa, spinach, black beans and pumpkin seeds. Chronic fatigue is sometimes greatly relieved by taking magnesium supplements.

SAMe (S-adenosylmethionine) has been effectively used to treat symptoms associated with fibromyalgia such as chronic arthritic pain and depression. Studies indicate that SAMe, which is naturally found in the body, may be lacking in some people suffering from fibromyalgia.

Do some research regarding supplements such as Capsicum, Coenzyme Q-10, Gingko and Melatonin. Studies have shown them to be very effective in relieving certain symptoms of fibromyalgia such as muscle pain and lack of sleep, which are very common to those suffering from the condition.

Fish oil, with its Omega-3 fatty acids is another supplement to consider when fighting fibromyalgia symptoms. It is well known for reducing inflammation and soothing stiffness and tender points.

The simple sugar, Ribose, may help relieve fibro pain and relax muscles. Your energy levels may increase by as much as 60% and help improve the fatigue associated with fibromyalgia.

Consider trialing brown seaweed extract as a supplement to relieve joint pain and stiffness. Research is now being conducted in this supplement as an answer to severe chronic pain.

Implementation

Revise your diet and exercise plans when thinking about taking supplements to relieve your fibromyalgia symptoms. Supplementation on its own is not a magic bullet and its benefits will be greater if a holistic approach is undertaken.

If you are determined to find answers for your pain and other symptoms, dietary supplementation could go a long way toward reducing the effects of your condition, as well as supporting you overall health.

Conclusion

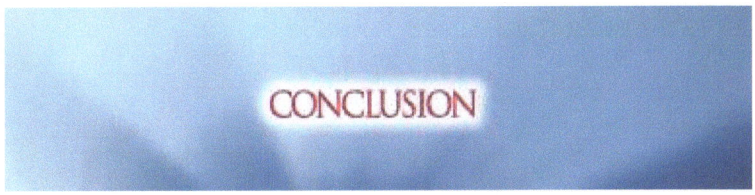

It is hoped that that those suffering from fibromyalgia realize that options exist to help improve their quality of life. It is not necessary or even noble to struggle with the effects of fibromyalgia without taking steps to alleviate them.

Pharmaceutical and natural health solutions are available. Public awareness of the condition is increasing; it is hoped that the understanding of non-sufferers will increase along with it!

Other Relevant Books by This Author

If you would like to read more relevant books about this topic, here is a list of the CreateSpace links, titles and descriptions from this author:

https://www.createspace.com/6853248

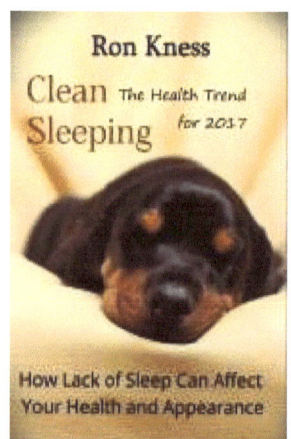

Clean Sleeping - The Health Trend for 2017: How Lack of Sleep Can Affect Your Health and Appearance

We want to be more energetic the next day . We also want to be more productive . And we want to get more sleep and of a better quality!

We can achieve ALL of these goals with the newest release from Ron Kness called Clean Sleeping - The Health Trend For 2017.

Based on these exciting teachings, you will learn about all the dramatic benefits of restful sleep and eating foods that help people sleep better.

This book is built around a very clear, concept: feel well rested.

It's not just about ways to get the maximum amount of restorative sleep. Having great sleeping habits is linked to eating healthy. This is because some foods are more conducive to sleeping well than others

In this book, we look at all of the ways you can improve your own sleeping habits, starting with calming the mind. This book will also look at the many other steps that can be taken to support this goal, from doing meditation before retiring for the night to taking a warm bath scented with an essential oil and listening to soft music. Even the choices you make about healthy eating and creating sleep-inducing bedroom environment can have an impact on your sleeping habits.

In Clean Sleeping - The Health Trend For 2017, we'll cover all the bases, giving you everything you need to know to get the maximum amount of quality sleep each night. It is the most important thing you can do for your overall physical and mental health.

The good news is that getting a good night's rest is totally doable ... we show you how!

https://www.createspace.com/6801309

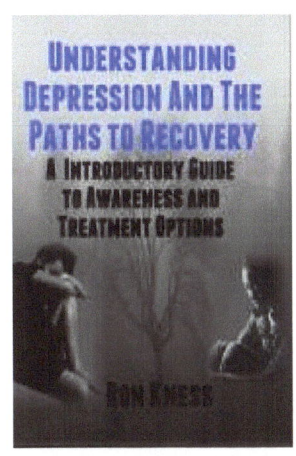

Understanding Depression and the Paths to Recovery: An Introductory Guide to Awareness and Treatment Options

While depression can hit during any time of year, winter in a cold climate and especially around the holidays, can be stressful and depressing for many people.

At any one time, 350 million people around the world suffer from some form of depression: Major Depressive Disorder, Postpartum Depression, PTSD, Seasonal Affective Disorder, Atypical Depression, and other depression conditions. It can literally cripple their lives and leave them non-functioning. Half of those suffering will not seek help.

Not seeking help only makes matters worse because when depression is not treated properly, it can lead to serious physical, emotional, and mental health issues, like:
- Long-term sadness
- Much reduced quality of life
- Lack of joy in living
- Extremely low levels of self-esteem
- Problems at work
- Low energy levels
- Skin, hair, and digestive system issues caused by chemical and hormonal responses to depression
- Body aches and pains, headaches and cramps
- Career and job failure
- Cognitive issues, including but not limited to difficulty making decisions, problems concentrating and focusing, and failed memory
- Insomnia or sleeping too much
- Significant weight gain or loss (not related to dieting)
- Reckless, harmful self-behavior like abusing alcohol, caffeine, food or drugs, compulsive gambling, and engaging in other physically risky behaviors
- Failed relationships, which can include emotional and physical pain inflicted on others
- Suicide
- And the list goes on and on

However, it doesn't have to be this way. Help is available.

In my book, you'll discover...
- Detailed and easy to understand definition of depression
- Risk factors that increase the likelihood that you will become depressed
- The different types of depression
- Symptoms and the diagnosis process and criteria
- How to choose the right doctor for diagnosis and treatment
- That total recovery is possible, even with the most severe depression cases
- The differences between major depression and simply feeling a temporary case of "the blues"
- Four depression conditions unique to women

- How limiting stress can boost your mood to beat and even prevent depression
- The differences of depression among various populations, such as men, women, and the elderly
- The major negative effects of untreated depression, including suicide
- Effective alternative treatment methods, including all natural methods and self-help home remedies
- And much, much more!

Don't you deserve a better quality of life, one where your mind and spirit are tranquil, healthy, and happy?

Depression is treatable - You can get better

Do not neglect this critical information a day longer! Get your copy today!

https://www.createspace.com/6923372

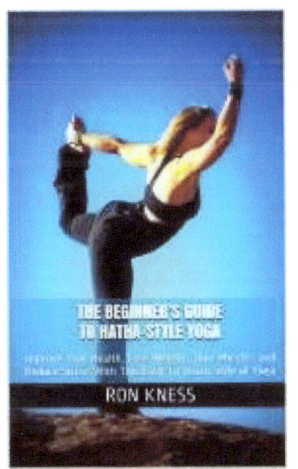

The Beginner's Guide to Hatha-Style Yoga: Improve Your Health, Lose Weight, Tone Muscles and Reduce Stress With This Easy-To-Learn Style of Yoga

We want there to be a calmness of in both our mind and spirit. We also want to be healthier as we age. And to accomplish both, we must learn to do the poses of Hatha yoga!

We can achieve ALL of these goals with the newest release from Ron Kness called "The Beginner's Guide To Hatha-Style Yoga".

Based on these exciting teachings, you will learn about all the dramatic benefits of doing Hatha yoga like improved health, weight loss, muscle toning and reducing stress, along with improved flexibility and balance.

This book is built around a very clear, concept: learn yoga and reap the benefits from doing this style of yoga - Hatha.

It's not just about learning how to do this easy-to-learn style of yoga. Having great overall health is linked to being in charge and making smart healthy lifestyle decisions. This is because learning how to do any style of yoga should be part of any healthy lifestyle.

In this book, we look at all of the ways you can improve your own overall health, starting with deciding to learn the poses and practice yoga. This book will also look at the many other steps that can be taken to support this goal, like viewing the suggested videos of poses used in Hatha yoga depending on the health benefit you want to gain.

The choices you make about joining a Hatha yoga class or learning it by yourself and doing it at home has a great impact on your overall health.

In "The Beginner's Guide To Hatha-Style Yoga", we'll cover all the bases, giving you everything you need to know to do this style of yoga that provides the health benefits mentioned.

Get your copy now and start improving your health tomorrow!

About the Author

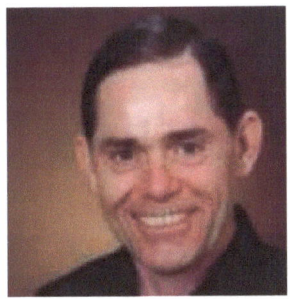

I have published over 125 books on Amazon for Kindle, CreateSpace and other publishing platforms.

While most of my books are on health and fitness in general, as I age (now 65) at the time of this writing) my topics of interest are geared toward aging baby boomers and older.

Besides my own writing, I also ghostwrite ebooks, books, reports, articles, blogs and do Kindle conversions for clients on a variety of topioo.

Today my wife and I are retired from our careers and live in Gold Canyon, AZ. I now write as a retirement business where you'll find me happily sitting in my office typing away on my laptop as I work on my next book or ghostwriting project . . . that is if we are not traveling on a cruise ship - our new-found mode of travel.

www.ingramcontent.com/pod-product-compliance
Lightning Source LLC
Chambersburg PA
CBHW050833290526
45792CB00001B/371